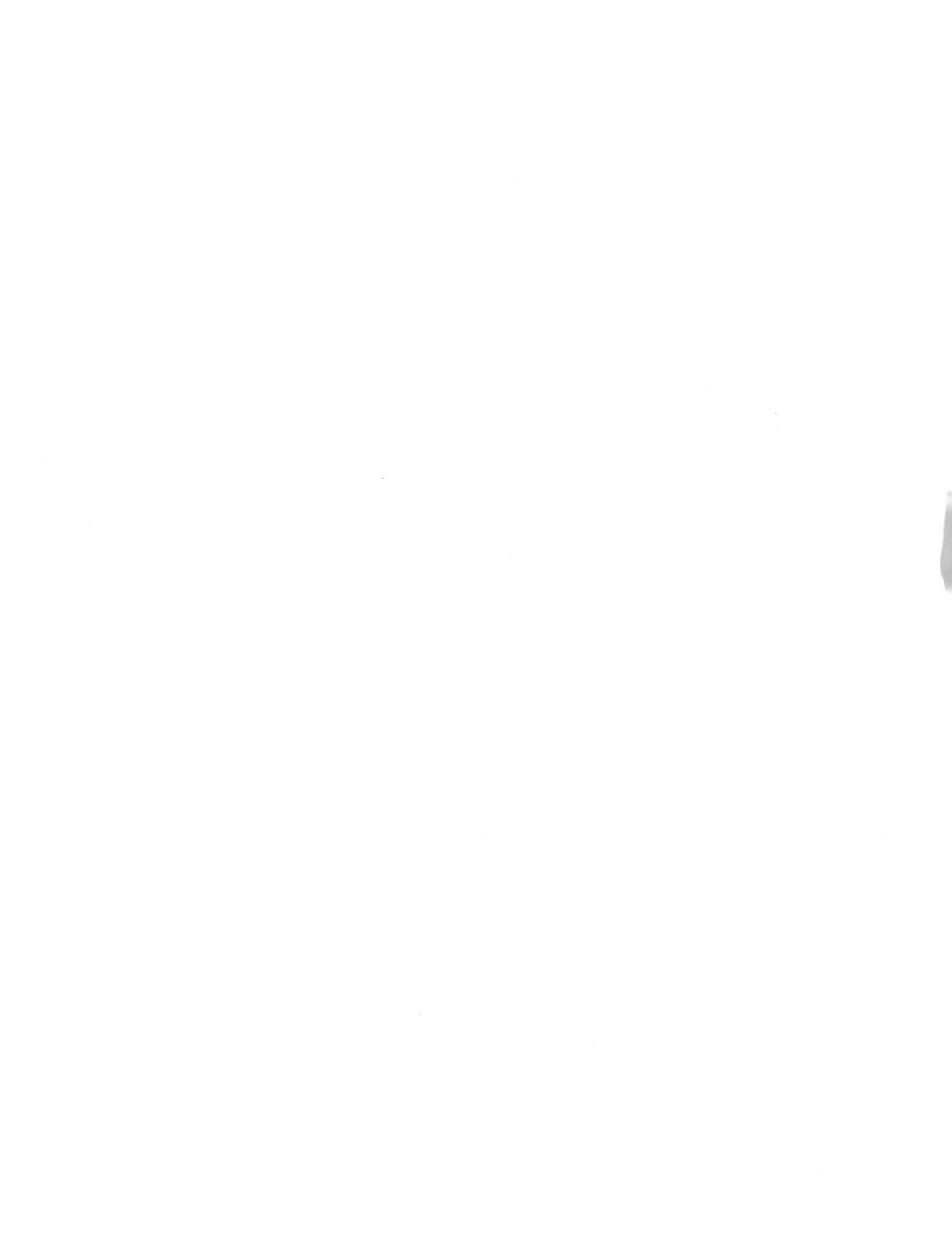

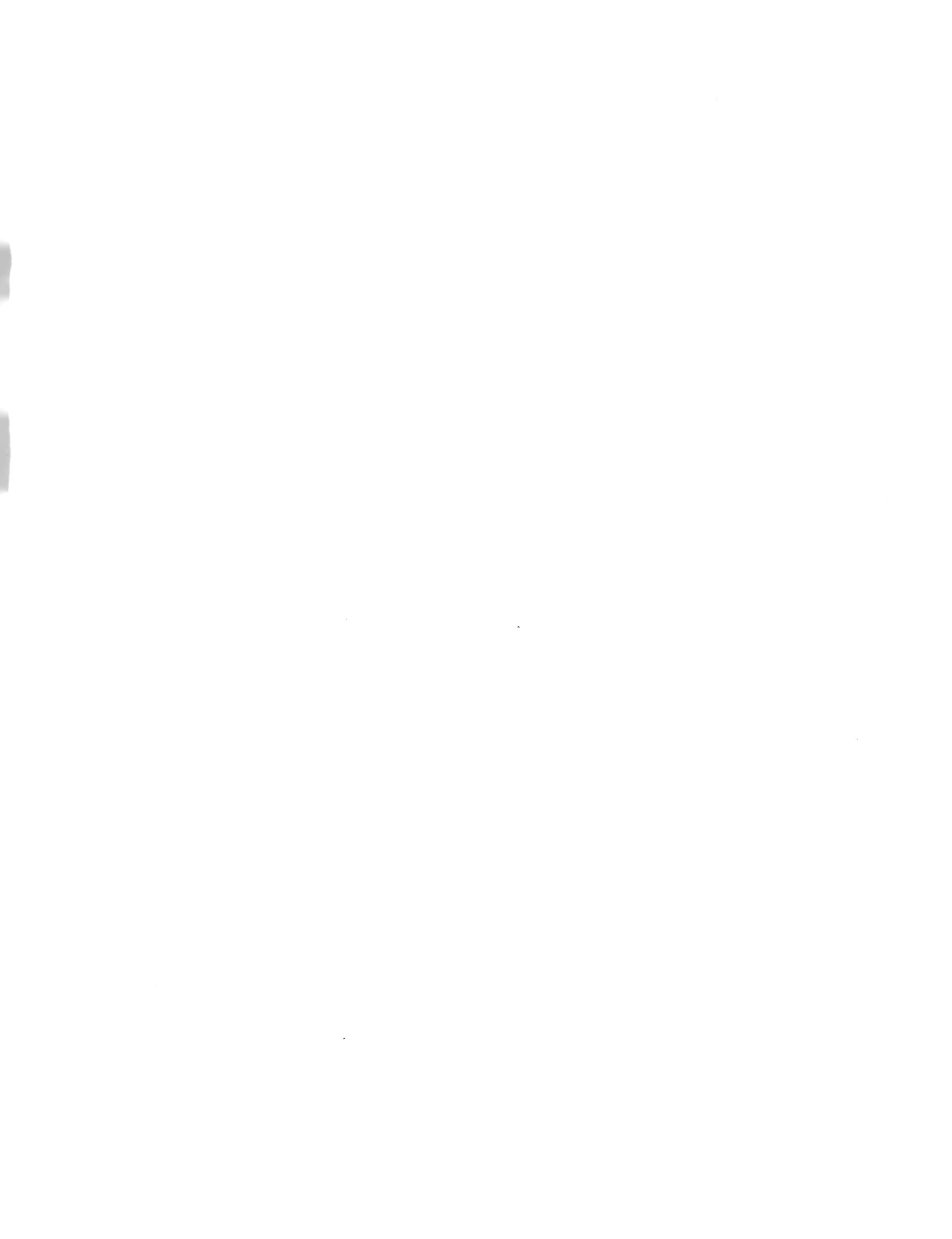

SLEEP WELL, WONDERFUL CHILD

BOOKS IN THE SAME SERIES

The Little Elephant Who Wants to Fall Asleep – A New Way of Getting Children to Sleep (Penguin Random House, 2016)
The Rabbit Who Wants to Fall Asleep – A New Way of Getting Children to Sleep (Penguin Random House, 2014)

OTHER BOOKS BY
CARL-JOHAN FORSSÉN EHRLIN

Goodwill Företagsekonomi 2 (co-writer) [Goodwill Business Economics] (2012)
Create Your Future! A Handbook in Leadership and Personal Development (2007)

A NEW WAY OF GETTING CHILDREN TO SLEEP

THE TRACTOR WHO WANTS TO FALL ASLEEP

CARL-JOHAN FORSSÉN EHRLIN
ILLUSTRATED BY SYDNEY HANSON

e.

EHRLIN PUBLISHING

ACKNOWLEDGEMENTS

Thank you to everyone who volunteered to be test readers and all others who
have helped make this book as sleep-promoting as possible.

Carl-Johan Forssén Ehrlin

The Tractor Who Wants to Fall Asleep is the third part in a series of sleep-promoting children's books.
It is also available as an e-book and audiobook.

VISIT US ONLINE!

www.carl-johan.com
www.ehrlinpublishing.com
facebook.com/carljohanforssenehrlin
facebook.com/therabbitwhowantstofallasleep

INSTRUCTIONS TO THE READER

Warning! Use this book with caution. It may cause drowsiness or an unintended catnap. And never read this book out loud close to someone driving any type of vehicle or engaged in any activity that requires wakefulness!

The author and the publisher very much hope your little one falls asleep, but make no guarantees and can take no responsibility for the outcome.

This book has been written to have a sleep-promoting effect, and therefore sometimes uses unusual language in order to help the child to relax and feel ready to sleep. Sometimes the child may need to hear the book a few times before he or she feels comfortable with the story and happily falls asleep.

To achieve the best results when you read this bedtime story, you should read it through to yourself first, so that you are familiar with the text and are more free to engage with the story when you read it to the child. I also recommend that you read through the tips at the end of the book in order to get the most out of this sleep-inducing bedtime story. *The Tractor Who Wants to Fall Asleep* is also available as an audiobook if you or your child would prefer that.

At certain points in the story, it is recommended that you adjust your tone of voice or yawn. Feel your way forward, and see what works best for your child.

- When the text is marked in **bold**, emphasise these words.
- When the text it marked with *italics,* try saying these words in a more soothing voice.
- Where it says [Name], feel free to insert your child's name.
- Where it says [Yawn], it would be a good idea to do so.

Good luck, and sleep well!

Carl-Johan Forssén Ehrlin

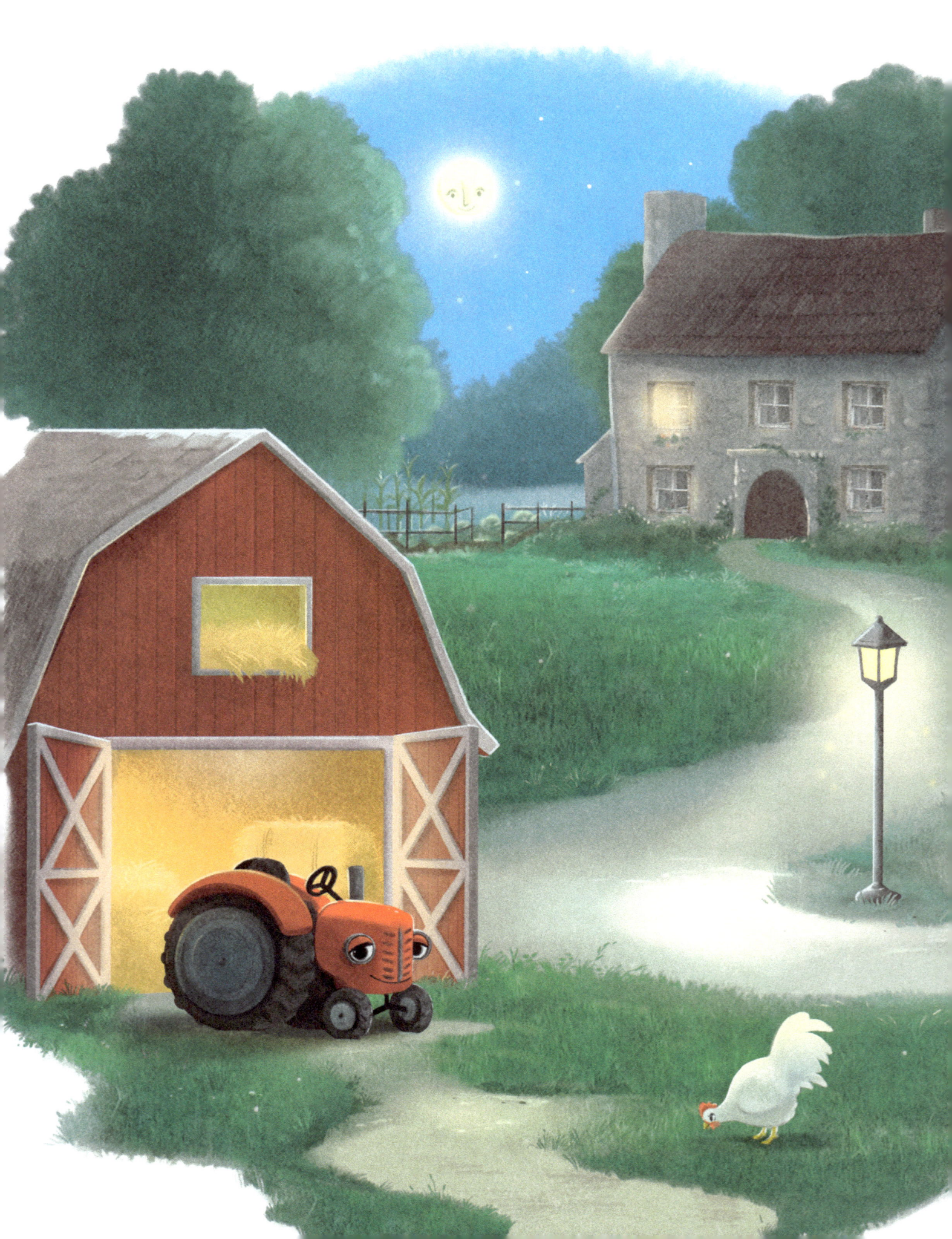

There is a little red tractor called Alex, who is exactly the same age as you. Alex the Tractor lives on a farm and likes to play and have fun, both alone and with friends. In this story you will follow Alex, as you go to see some of Alex's lovely friends.

In the evening Alex the Tractor wants to fall fast asleep, but doesn't always succeed. Alex sometimes lies down and thinks about other things, forgetting everything else except **remembering to fall asleep** *and just letting it happen.*

The tractor's best friend, Farmer Gotobed, finds it very easy to fall asleep, a bit like you soon will too. Now Farmer Gotobed has already gone to bed and is sleeping soundly in his soft, cosy bed. He said: "Goodnight" before **falling asleep almost straight away** when listening to a *sleepy story.* Alex is wondering when you, just like Farmer Gotobed, **are going to fall asleep to this story**, **now**, or in a little while.

Alex the Tractor thinks: "I've got friends who can tell me what they do to fall asleep, and teach me how I can **be all lovely and sleepy too**, *and just fall asleep.* Let's go and talk to them."

Alex the Tractor leaves the barn, looks at you and says: "When you come with me in the story, [Name], you too will learn how easy it can be to, **feel so relaxed and sleepy in the evening**."

Together you set off on a journey that will help you to, **always be able to**, **fall sound asleep in the evening**.

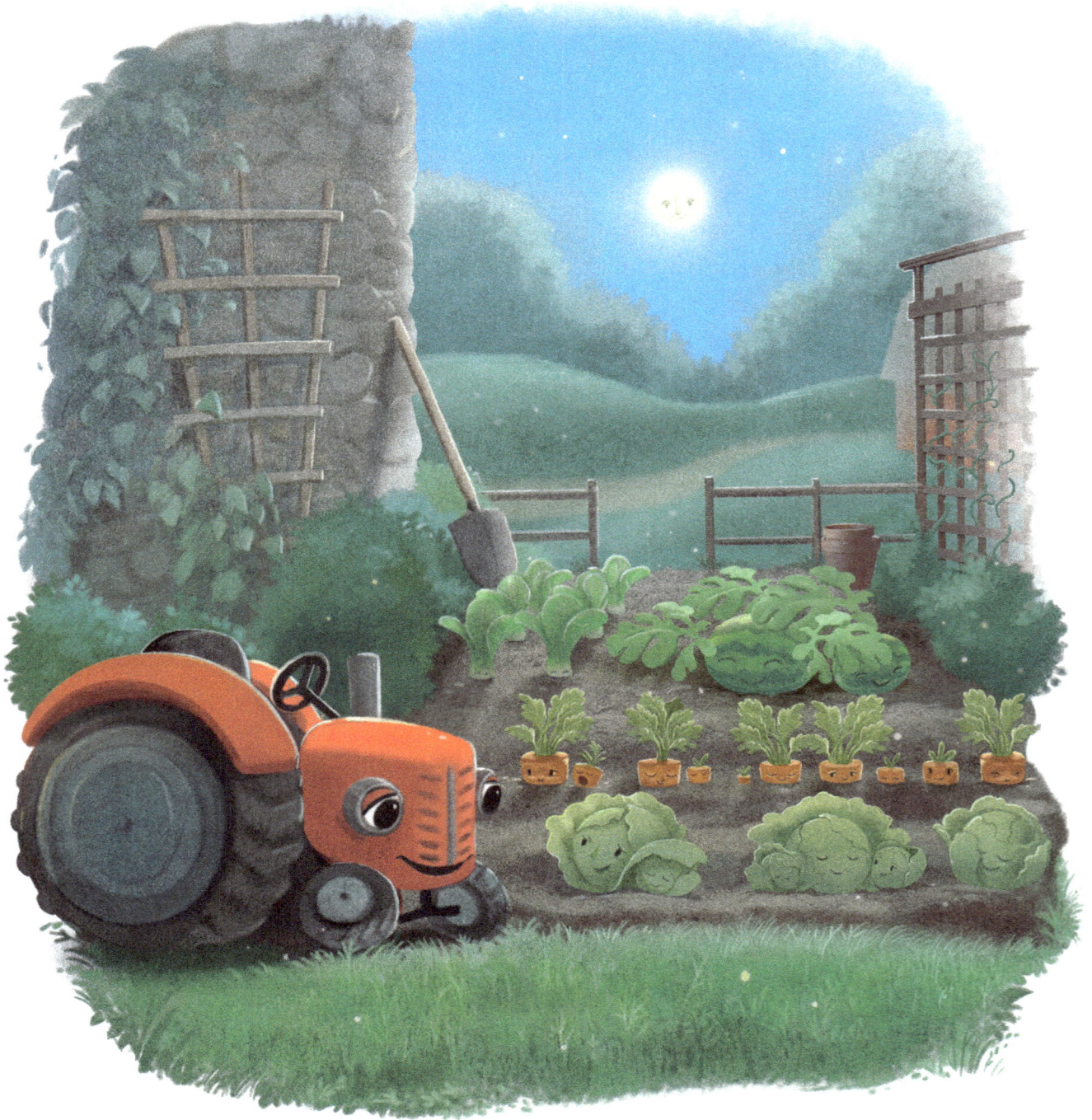

When you and Alex go round the back of the house where Farmer Gotobed is, **already lying fast asleep**, you come to the sleep inducing vegetable patch, where the farmer grows lots of **sleepy** vegetables. This is where Yawning Carrot lives with her little carrots, and Lazy Lettuce with her baby lettuce. They look at you *and yawn*. [Yawn]

They look so calm and relaxed as they just sit there letting everything else just fade away. They're living in this moment, in a very sleepy way. Alex the Tractor asks gently what they do to help them fall sound asleep in the evening.

Lazy Lettuce replies in a sleepy voice: "*When my baby lettuce and I are* **going to sleep**, *my baby lettuce or I try to stay awake, but the more I try to stay awake,* **the more tired I become**, **right now.** *Which always makes me fall asleep.*" [Yawn]

Yawning Carrot says: "The same thing happens to me. When evening comes, and I try to do anything else except **fall asleep straight away**, I then get more and more tired and the more tired I get, **the tireder you become**, [Name], *the easier it is to fall asleep. And then I ... fall asleep ... when ...*"

Yawning Carrot falls asleep in the middle of the sentence, before the story ends. Since this story will help both you and Alex the Tractor to **fall fast asleep**, you can do exactly the same as Yawning Carrot and, **just let your eyelids close** and look at the insides of your eyelids now that you want to, **close your eyes now**, *and just fall asleep.*

Alex the Tractor says to you: "We're just like these vegetables. Wherever we are, we grow and get big. And as we do, we feel safe and secure. The sort of security that makes me ready to **let the story help me to sleep**. To sleep soundly all night through. To be kind to other people, grownups and children alike, and to feel grateful that I am alive and will be *sleeping soundly very soon.*"

Now everyone in the vegetable patch has fallen asleep, and together with Alex the Tractor you creep away carefully, so that all the vegetables and **you, can sleep soundly**.

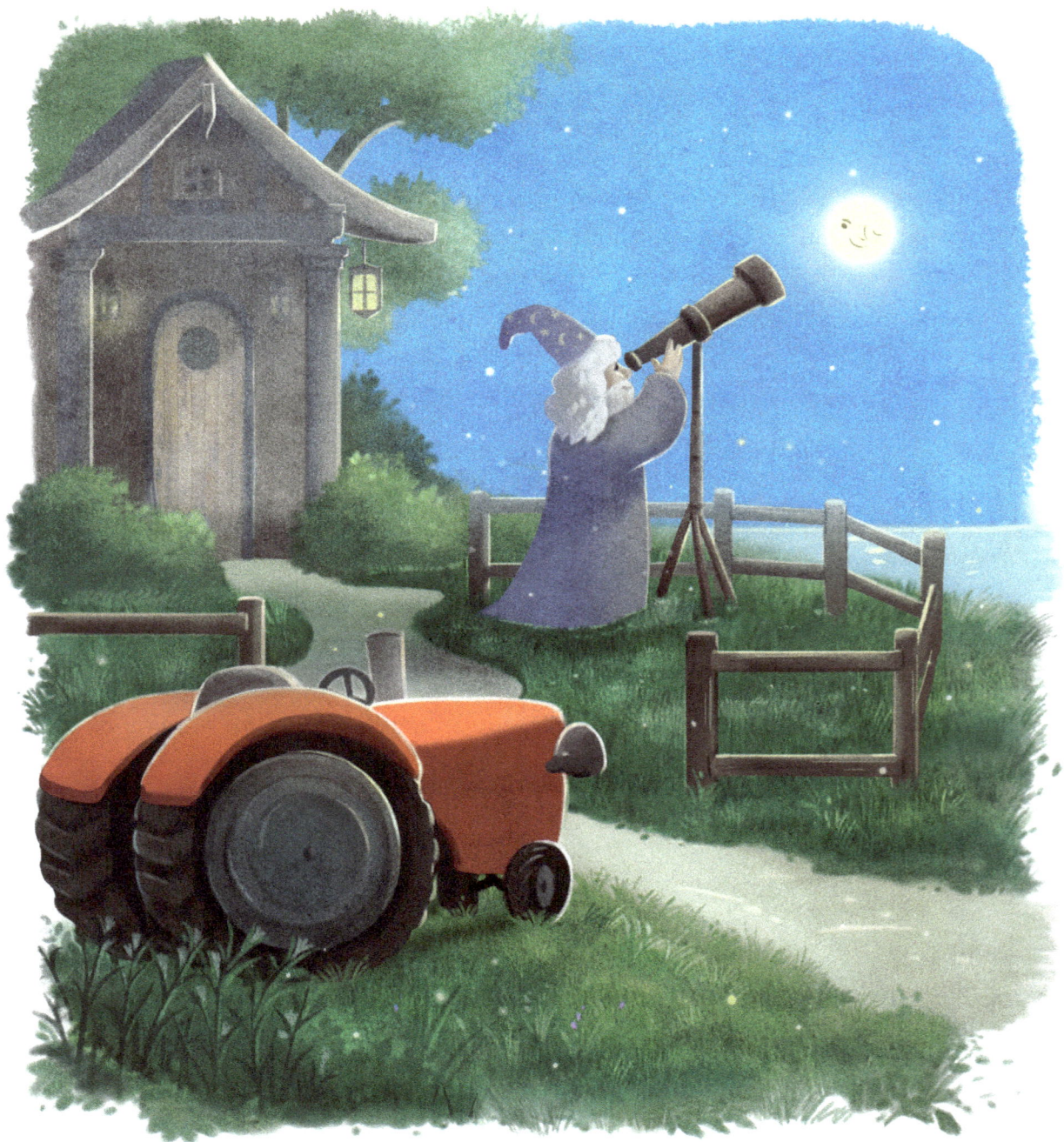

Alex the Tractor and you carry on across a meadow, and reach the house where Uncle Yawn lives. He always has good advice, and has helped lots and lots of children, **to sleep**. Uncle Yawn is standing outside the house with his sleepy pyjamas on, looking at the beautiful sky through a telescope. He looks a bit tired, and Alex the Tractor wonders what's *making him so tired, so so tired*.

Uncle Yawn says: "I'm tired, but this evening it's not that easy to fall asleep. However, to make myself **really tired** I look through my telescope at all the sleepy stars, and start counting them. For every star I count I also get **more and more tired**, **more and more tired**. We can start counting stars together, but I have to tell you – I usually **fall asleep really quickly** when I do that, nearly always **before I've finished counting**."

Alex the Tractor yawns and starts feeling tired at the very thought of you both falling asleep as you count the stars. [Yawn] You start counting stars together, and I wonder how many you'll manage to count before **you fall asleep** [Name].

One star.
Two stars, your eyelids want to close.
Three stars, so tired.
Four stars. [Yawn]
Five stars, tired, oh so tired [Name].
Six stars, sleepy stars.
Seven stars, twice as tired.
Eight stars, even more tired.
Nine stars, want to sleep, so tired.
And ten stars, really tired, and now all the stars are asleep.

"I need to go to bed now, but you can carry on counting sleeping stars until you too are fast asleep soon," Uncle Yawn says, also **very tired now**, *and falling asleep soon.*

Alex the Tractor thanks Uncle Yawn and you leave, full of **a sleepy feeling** *as you slowly roll on along the road carrying you down into sleep.*

Alex the Tractor and **you are tireder now**, as you carry on along the journey that will make both of you **fall asleep**. You reach the calm water where Ellen the Elephant is *lying down comfortably, relaxing* on the beach.

[Yawn] "Hello, Ellen," Alex says while yawning. "What do you do to **fall sound asleep in the evening now**."

"Daddy Elephant has taught me what to do, to just close my eyes and fall asleep in the evening. I'll teach you how **you can fall asleep easily now** [Name]," Ellen the Elephant says.

She takes a small boat made of bark, puts it in the water and says: "Think of all the things that are not making you **fall asleep right now**, all the thoughts and feelings that are swirling round inside you. Even all the things you'd like to do instead of, **fall asleep now**. Put all those thoughts and feelings on this boat, and when **you do that now**, I want you to blink a few times with your eyes, which will soon be closed."

Alex the Tractor thinks for a little while, then Alex and you decide to do as Ellen the Elephant suggests. You think about putting all the reasons why you're not asleep, on the boat. All the thoughts and feelings you have, all the things that used to be an excuse for not **falling fast asleep**. And now that you feel ready to get rid of all of that, you blink your eyes a few times, and your heavy eyelids close again, and you just want to keep them closed.

Ellen the Elephant gently pushes the bark-boat with her trunk, and says: "*Now, as the boat with all your thoughts and feelings glides further and further out into the water, you feel a big change inside you. You're free from thoughts and worries, and just let go and fall asleep. You feel light and free, light and free.*"

Alex the Tractor agrees with Ellen the Elephant: "*Yes, that's right, now that all my thoughts and feelings have drifted off on the boat, I am light and free, and my body feels all nice and heavy and I can fall asleep whenever I like.*" [Yawn]

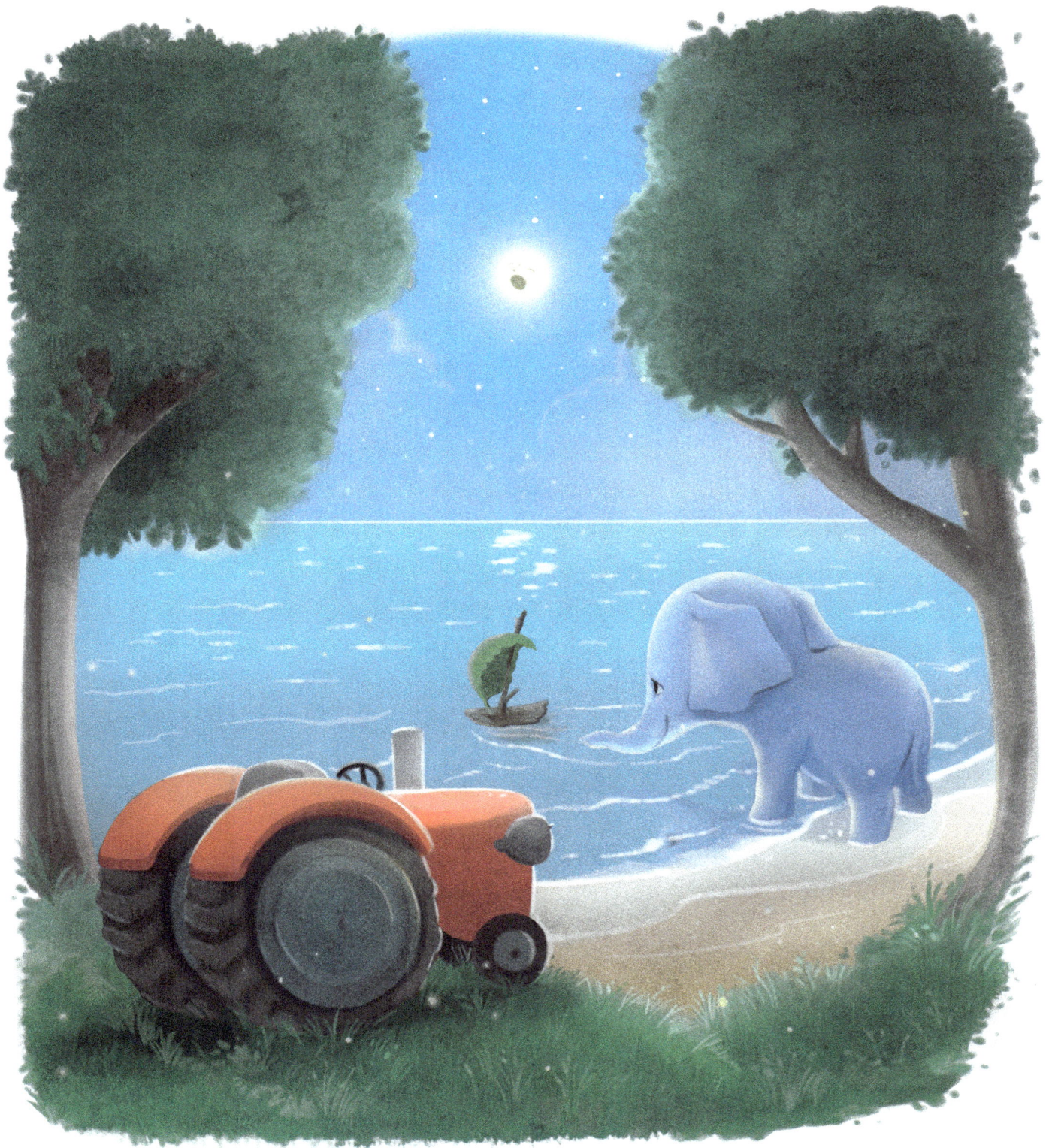

"The further out into the water the boat glides, the smaller and smaller it gets, and **you get more and more relaxed, and more and more ready to fall asleep**. *The boat is getting smaller and smaller, soon you can't even see it anymore, leaving you behind, ready to fall asleep now,*" Ellen the Elephant says softly.

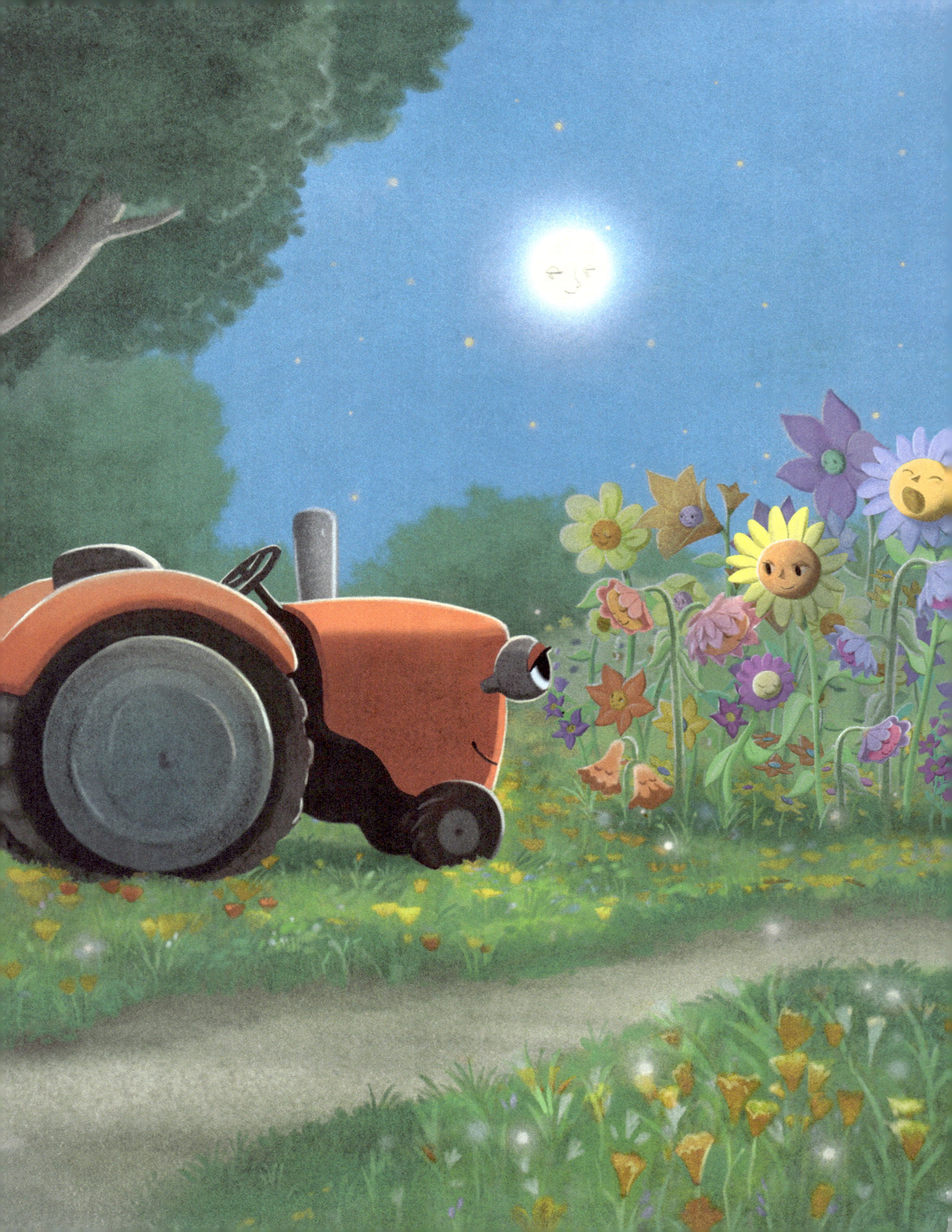

Alex the Tractor is also feeling very tired now, and starts to head home to, **fall asleep and sleep soundly all night long**, just like you, [Name].

In a rolling meadow beside the road, Alex the Tractor sees some beautiful flowers. They look different, they have different names, and are all the colours of the rainbow. They live together in harmony, and they look **calm**, **peaceful and tired**, **right now**.

Alex the Tractor stops by the meadow and asks: "Hello, flowers, what do you do to **fall asleep now**?"

"Shhh. We're lulling ourselves to sleep. We have to whisper, some of us have already fallen asleep," says the flower, Sleepy Sara. *"There are so many of us who want to fall asleep now, and more and more are falling asleep all the time. [Yawn] I'll tell you what we do to fall asleep."*

"First you need to lie down, [Name], and *let your whole body go soft,*" Sleepy Sara says. As she asks you to do this, more flowers fall asleep around her. They're just as beautiful and calm as you are now.

"When **you relax**, *the wind will slowly and sleepily take care of you. Let the wind rock you back and forth, slowly back and forth, so sleepily, so lovely."*

Alex the Tractor and you decide to close your eyes and *relax. You let yourself slowly and sleepily be rocked to sleep now. Just slowly and sleepily be rocked to sleep, now. The wind carries you back and forth, back and forth. Slowly and gently. So lovely, just to be rocked to sleep now.*

Now Alex the Tractor and you are very tired. You thank Sleepy Sara for her help and roll slowly on, heading for home to go to sleep now.

A few sleepy moments later you and Alex the Tractor meet a friend who is *slowly* walking along the road with his mummy. It's the tired little boy Half-Asleep Leon and his mummy, who are going for a walk and who will soon be sound asleep in his bed. Half-Asleep Leon is just your age, and he's just as tired as you, [Name], and is going to **be, even more tired very soon**.

"Hello, Half-Asleep Leon. What do you do to fall fast asleep?" Alex the Tractor asks gently.

"My parents have taught me how to fall asleep, so that **I fall asleep really easily every evening**," Half-Asleep Leon replies, and goes on: "Mummy can teach you too, how to fall asleep and sleep soundly where **you are going to sleep now**, **all night through**, and we'll soon be falling fast asleep together."

Half-Asleep Leon's mummy says to you: "If I tell you, you have to promise to lie down and do as I say."

Because you both, **want to fall asleep, you do that now**. You lie down and listen to the story and let it rock you to sleep.

Leon's sleepy mummy says: "*You can feel your eyelids getting heavier and heavier, as you get more and more relaxed.*"

"*Imagine that your eyelids just want to close, and shut your eyes, just close and shut your eyes, and the more you close your eyes, the more you want to fall asleep now. Even if you don't want to close your eyes right now to fall asleep, the more you don't want to, the more your eyes close. It feels completely natural and your eyes just get more and more tired the more you think about it.*"

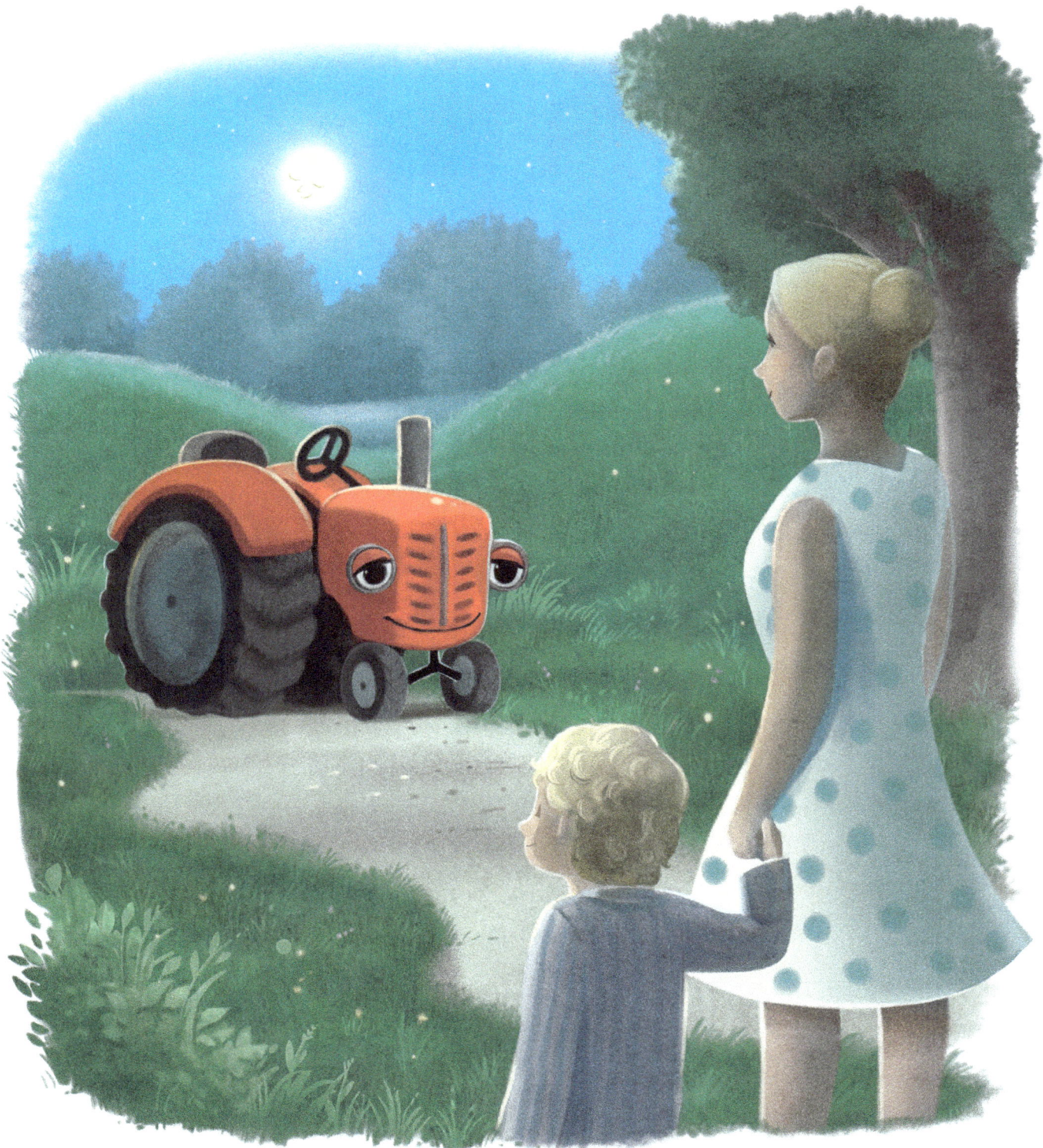

Half-Asleep Leon, who has made himself all comfy, starts to fall asleep, and his eyelids close as softly as yours are too, now. Now Leon has fallen asleep and you will do too, very soon. [Yawn]

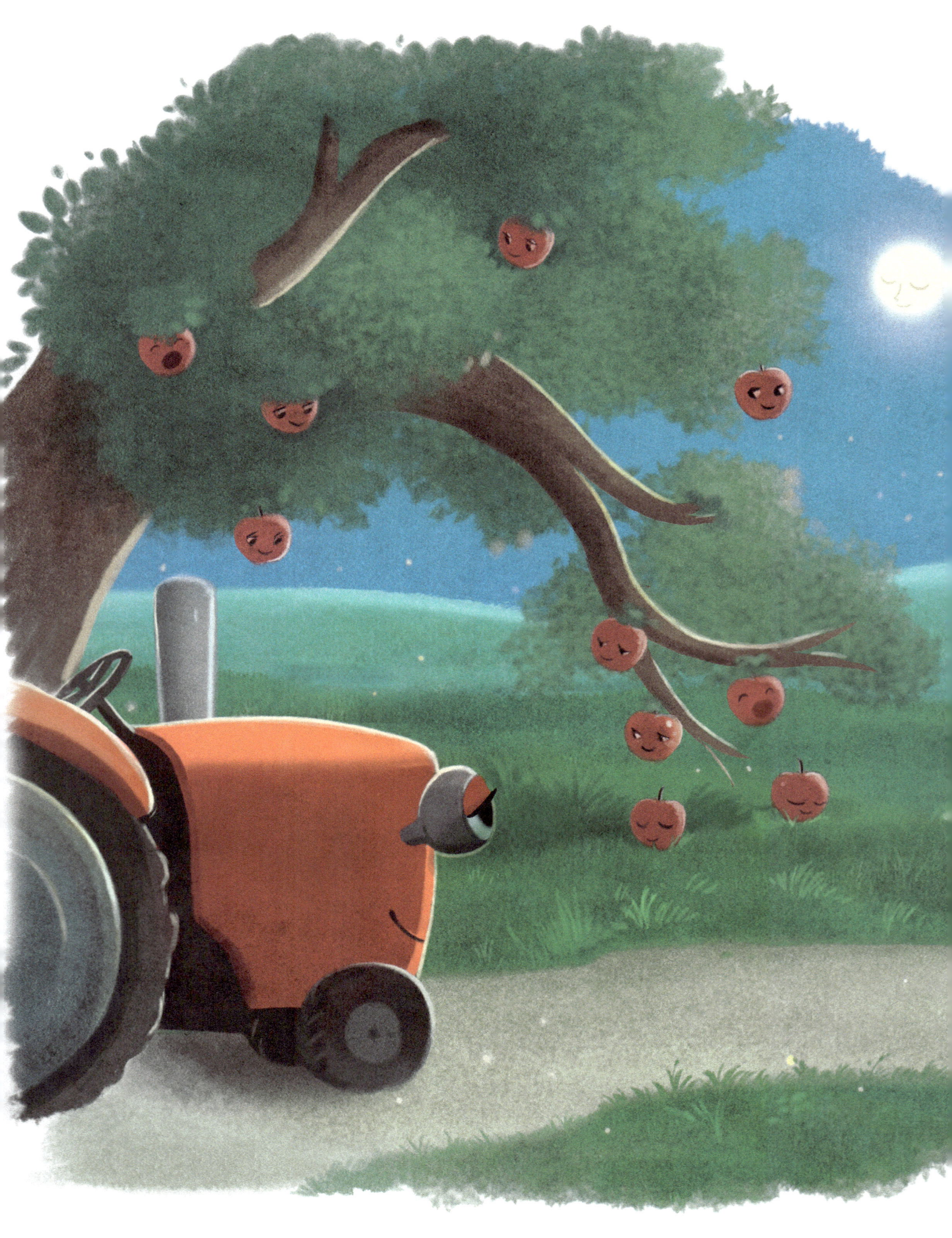

Slowly you and Alex the Tractor make your way further along the road. [Yawn]

When you reach the Tired Tree *with the sleepy apples*, you stop, to find out what the apples do to **fall asleep**.

"Hello, sleepy apples," Alex says in a tired voice.

"Hello, Alex the Tractor," the apples reply slowly, **about to fall asleep**.

"What do you do to fall asleep?" Alex wonders.

"We like landing on the soft ground that's our bed, and resting," the sleepy apples reply.

They go on explaining, and you listen: "There comes a time, like now, when we decide to fall asleep. We hang on our branch, and when we feel ready, the branch slowly reaches down to the ground and we let go of it, so we can *land nice and softly on our bed, in a lovely sleepy way.* We can do it together, *land nice and softly on our bed now.* When you feel ready, you can imagine that you're like us apples all **ready, to fall asleep now**."

You and Alex the Tractor feel ready to do the same as the apples, who are just about to let go of the branch or their parent's arms, land softly and **fall fast asleep, all night through**.

Slowly, slowly the sleepy apples and you let go and land in sleep, and sleep soundly all night through.

The apples land nice and softly on the ground, like you in your bed [Name], *and now you're all fast asleep together.*

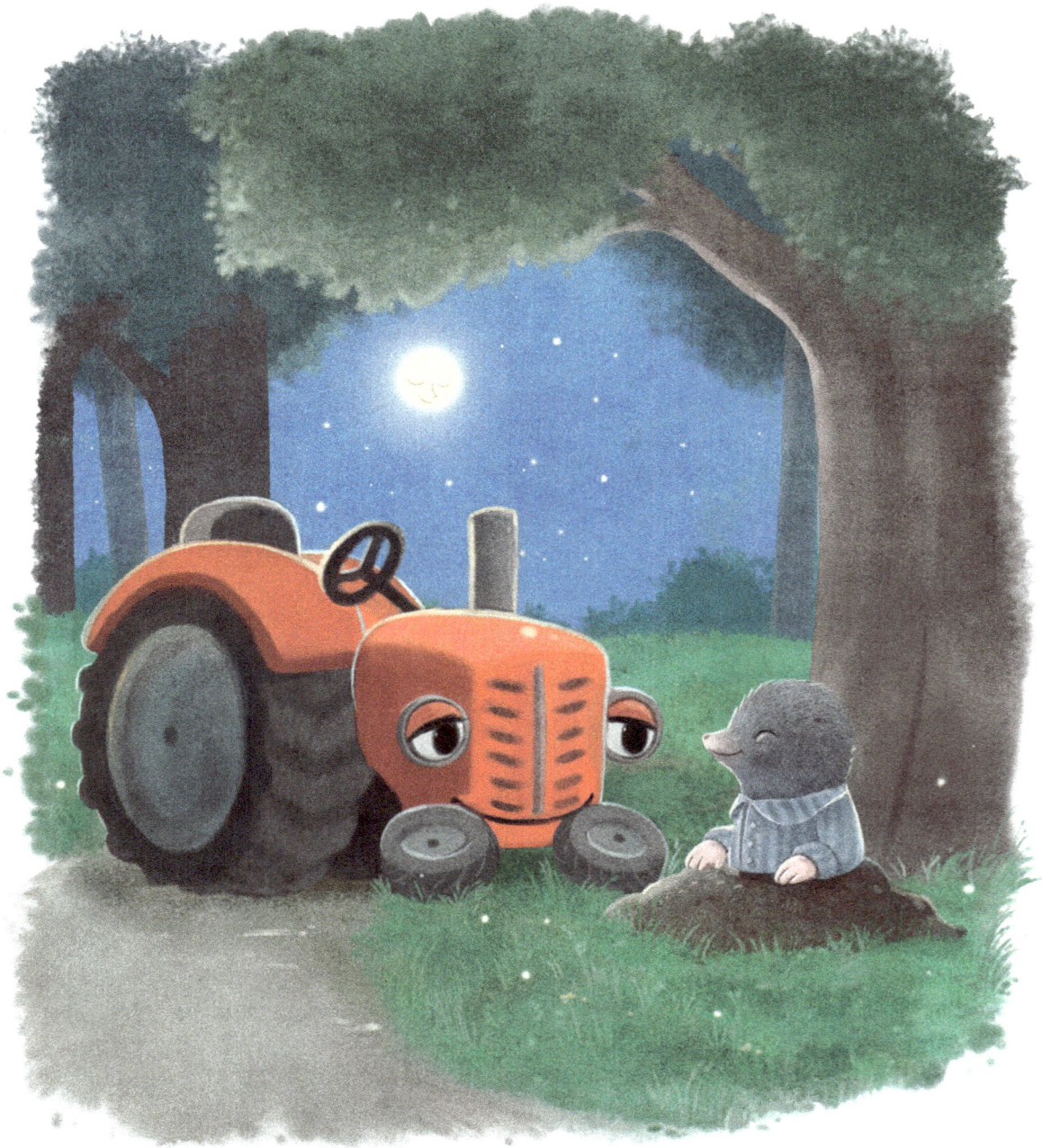

Just like you, Alex the Tractor is really tired, and wants to fall sound asleep. Slowly you make your way home, more and more tired, more and more tired. [Yawn]

On this particular evening, Snoozy Mole is sitting at his hole in the ground when Alex the Tractor rolls past.

Snoozy Mole says to Alex, very sleepily: "*I'm trying to get to sleep, and I know I'm about to fall asleep soon, really soon.*"

Snoozy Mole says he wants to teach Alex the Tractor and you [Name], how **to fall asleep all on your own**. You're very grateful, and ask what you have to do to, **fall fast asleep now**.

In his comforting voice, Snoozy Mole says: "**If you do this, you'll fall asleep**. *Lie down comfortably on your soft and really sleepy pillow as you let your head rest on it, all night. You'll sleep really well now, my friend.*"

Deep down, you know that it's true – **you're going to sleep well, all night through**.

Snoozy Mole goes on: "*Let your hands and arms lie next to your body. Let your arms feel heavy and* ...

... **tired, let your legs sink cosily into your bed, and** ...

... **just relax**. *Your breathing is getting calmer and calmer, you feel more and more ready to* ...

... **fall asleep now**. *Your whole body is getting heavier and heavier, heavier and heavier as you, now follow what I'm saying to you and* ...

... **fall fast asleep** *in your bed.*"

You both feel really tired now, and want to set off slowly towards dreamland.

You and Alex the Tractor carry on homewards, *very slowly and yawning a lot. You're both so tired that you just want to go to sleep now.* [Yawn] Alex the Tractor thinks about all the things you've been told by your friends, about how they fall asleep and how easy it is to make use of what they've said in order to fall fast asleep in the evening.

At the edge of the forest Alex the Tractor sees Roger the Rabbit, who really is extremely tired. He's on his way home from seeing Uncle Yawn, and will soon be at home in his lovely bed.

"Hello, Roger the Rabbit, I can see that you're about to fall asleep," Alex the Tractor says.

Roger the Rabbit is so tired that you can hardly hear what he says when he whispers: *"Come with me for the last part of my walk home. It will make you really tired. If you decide to imitate my slow pace and close your eyes, it will mean you choose to sleep really well, choosing to sleep really well now."*

Alex the Tractor slows down and rolls along at the same slow pace as Roger the Rabbit. It goes very slowly, and Alex the Tractor just wants to **close your eyes and fall asleep**, *just like Roger the Rabbit and you.*

When you reach Roger the Rabbit's house, he's so tired that he can hardly open the door, he's so tired. [Yawn] *Alex the Tractor says: "Goodnight," and tries to roll slowly homeward, even though you are both really tired now.*

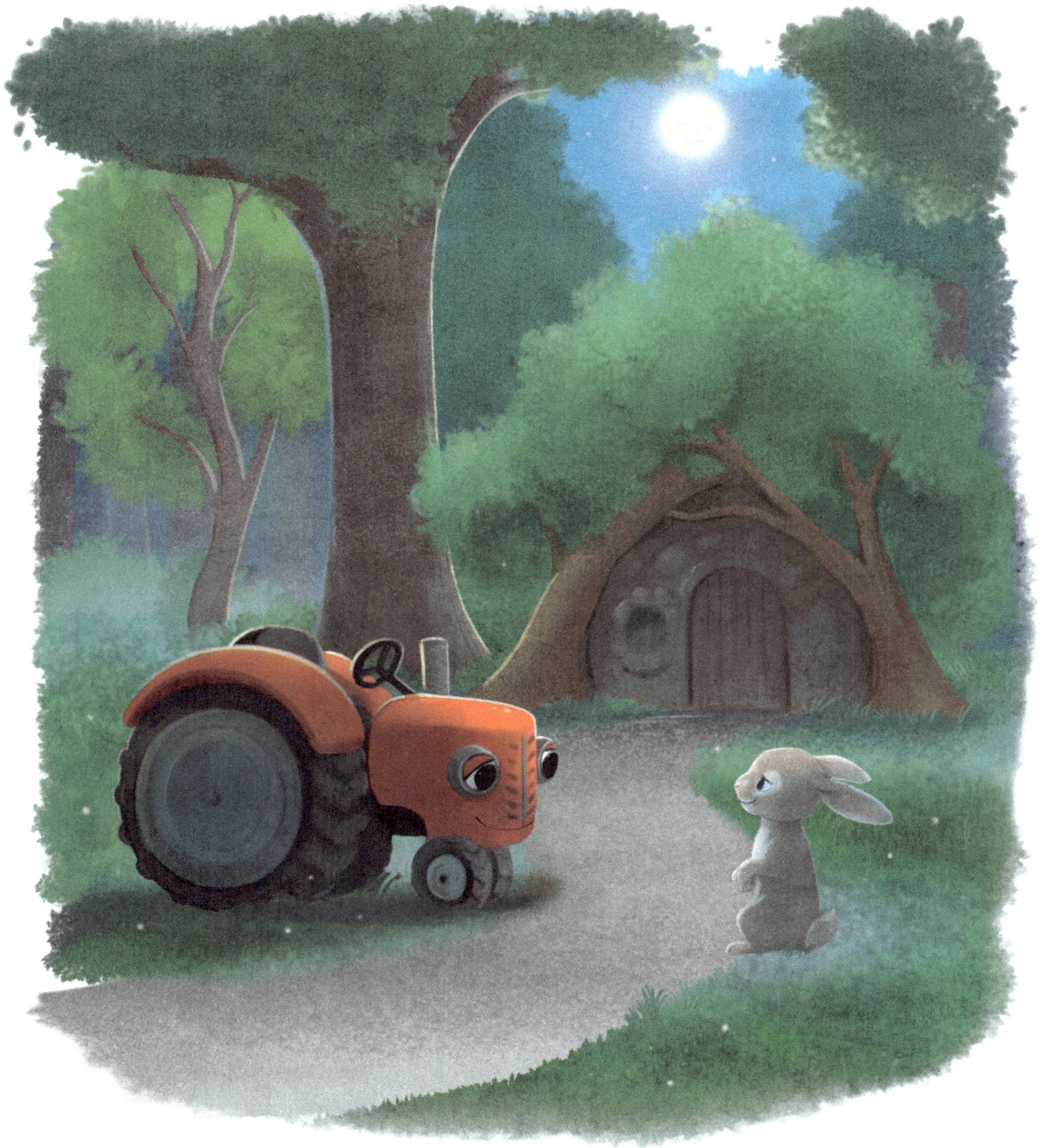

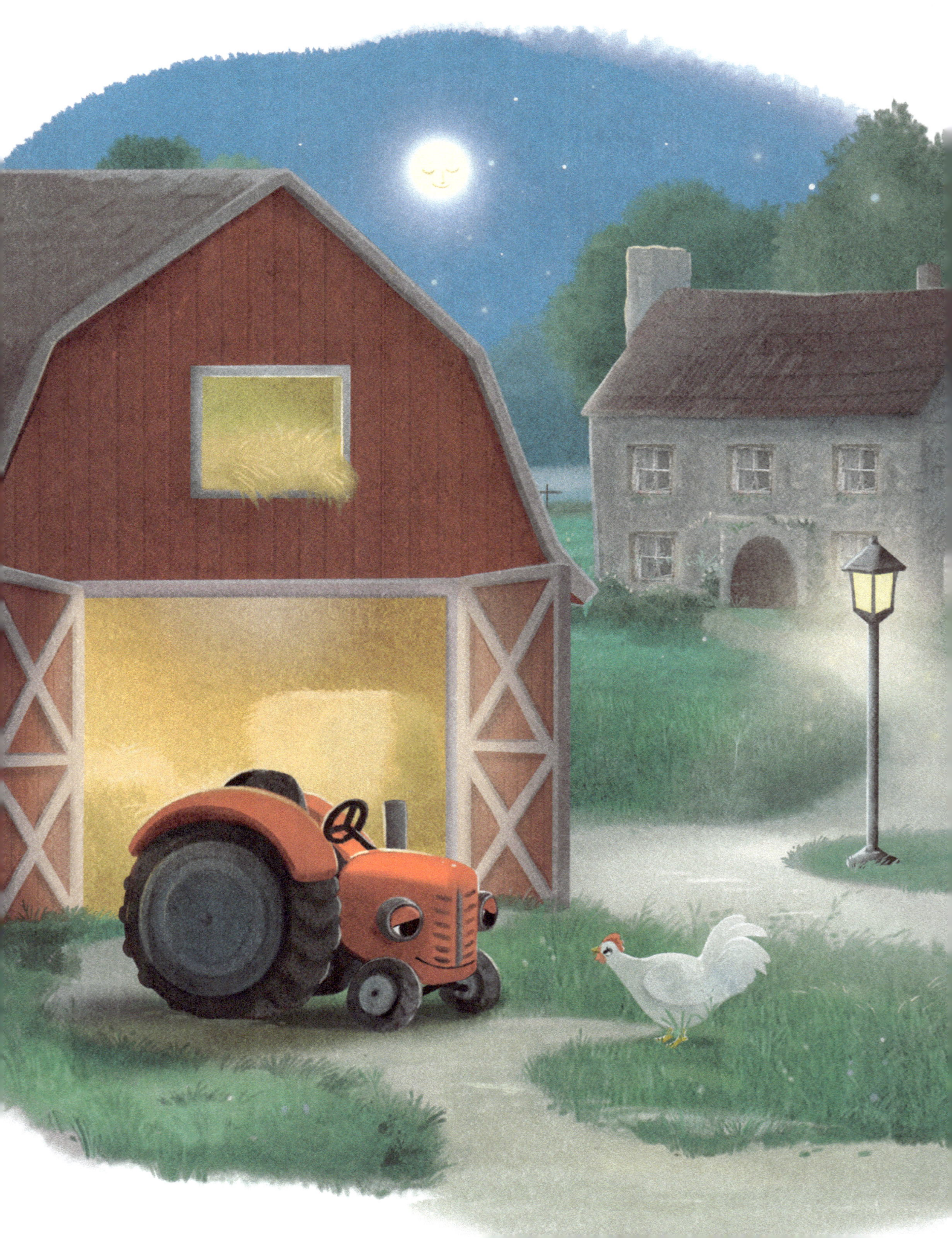

Alex the Tractor rolls into the farmyard, and will soon be back in the barn to fall fast asleep, every night. Alex and you are extremely tired now.

In front of the barn waits the tiredest animal on the farm, Hilda the Hen. Everyone always says that Hilda the Hen is the most tired out of everyone, and now she's thinking of you, because you're just as tired.

When Alex the Tractor is home again, all calm and cosy inside, the very tired Hilda says to you: **"At last, it's time to fall asleep.** I've been waiting for you to get back, so I can fall fast asleep now with your help."

Hilda, the very tiredest hen of them all, goes on slowly: "Every time I see you roll past on your sleepy wheels, or hear this story, **I know it's time to sleep.** *I usually watch your tractor wheels as they slow down, and then I slow down too and become more relaxed.* [Yawn] If you park in the barn, I'll show you what I mean."

Alex the Tractor starts to reverse into the barn. *As the tractor slows down, gently slows down, Alex notices that Hilda, the tiredest hen of them all, watches the wheels as they turn more and more slowly. At the same time, Alex the Tractor sees both you and Hilda the Hen getting tireder and tireder.*

Sleepier and sleepier, the slower they go.
Sleepier and sleepier, slowly they go, now. [Yawn]

As Alex the Tractor slows down more and more, and then stops altogether, you and Hilda the Hen both fall into a deep sleep, and sleep soundly all night through. Oh, how lovely it is to fall asleep now, you think and feel in your entire body.

Alex the Tractor settles down in bed, and is **now, very tired**. [Yawn] Alex thinks about all the good things your friends have said. *About what they do to help them relax and fall sound asleep in the evening,* **when it now, is time to fall asleep**.

Alex remembers how they all relax so easily each evening, when they **decide to fall asleep**, and how easy it is to **fall asleep now**.

Alex the Tractor is very tired after the drive, and can feel that **you too will fall asleep very soon**. Alex wonders which one of you will fall asleep first, you or Alex, seeing as you're both **really tired now**.

"Tonight I'm going to dream about things that will help me understand that I'm fine just the way I am, and that I can do far more things than I can imagine, like falling fast asleep in the evening, every evening from now on," Alex whispers in a sleepy voice.

Alex the Tractor is lying down on the comfy bed and just relaxes, eyes closed, ready to fall asleep. Alex feels like saying goodnight to you, even if you might already be asleep now.

You feel confident that you will be able to go to sleep all on your own, even if the person reading the story might soon leave the room.

Your eyelids droop, slowly and sleepily, and with your eyes closed you say "Goodnight" to each other, and fall into a lovely deep sleep. [Yawn]

Sleep well, wonderful child.

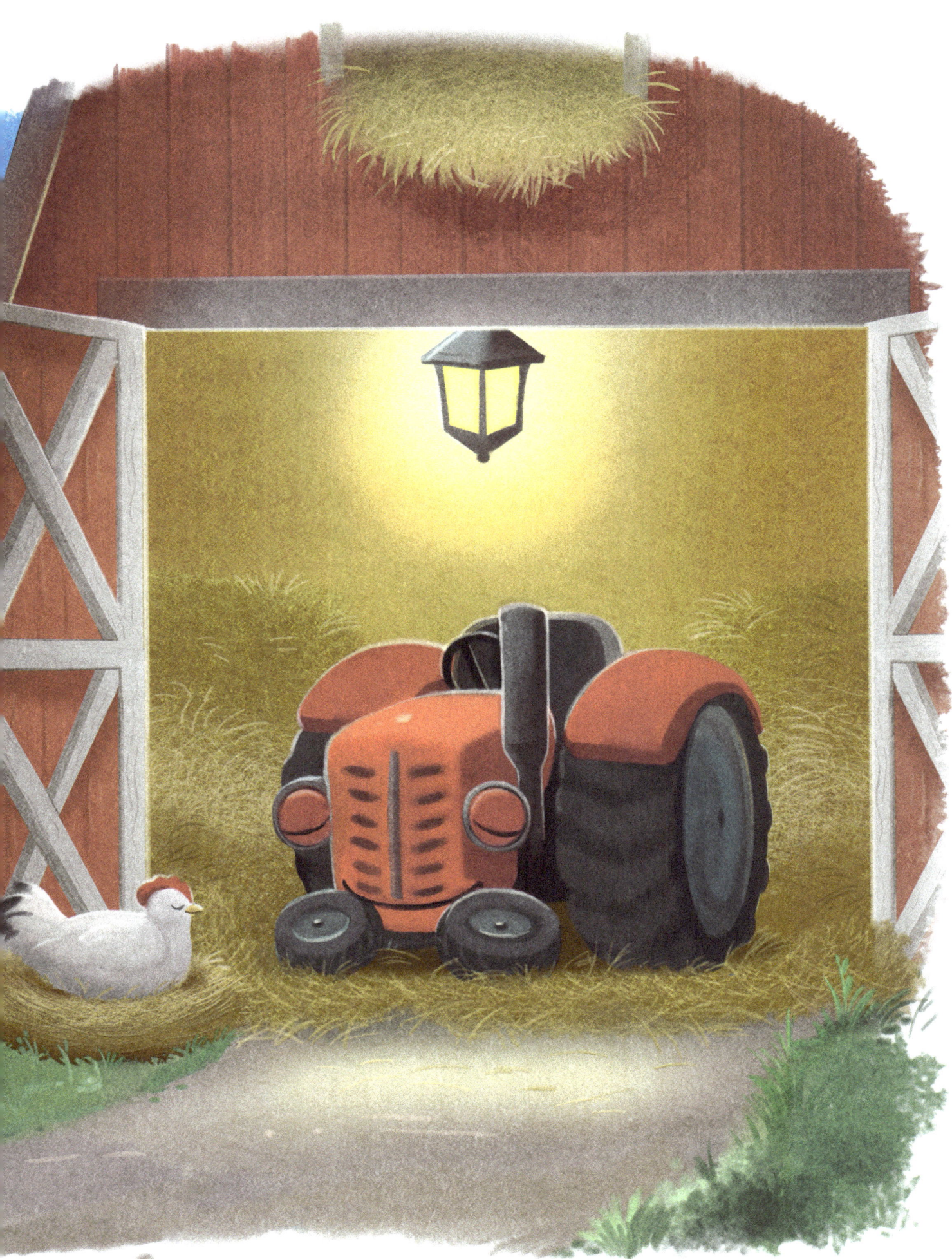

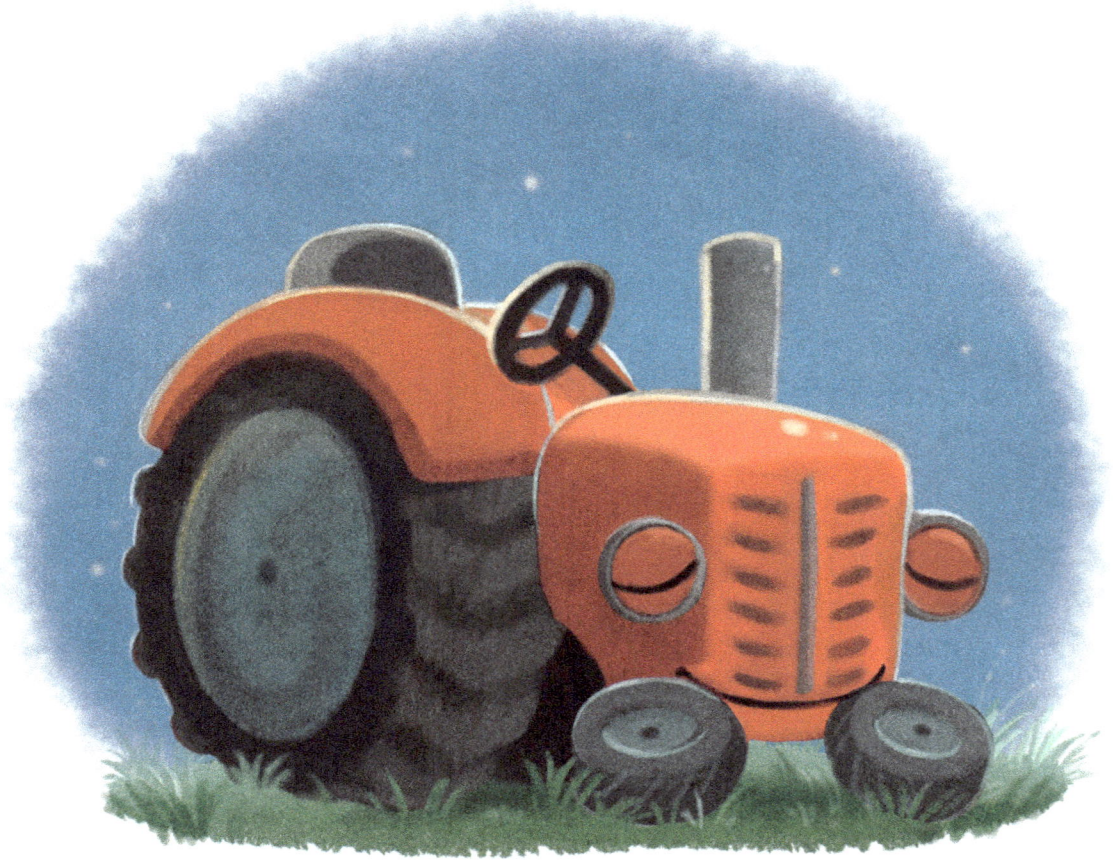

TIPS FROM THE AUTHOR

The way you choose to introduce my sleep-inducing books to the child can have a decisive effect on how well you will succeed. Because all children are different, there's no universal solution to get the child to want to listen to the story in order to sleep well. Lots of parents have said they've told the child that it's a magical book that you can only read in the evening, because it makes you fall asleep. Some parents have chosen to let the child look through the book on his or her own during the day and talk about the pictures, and then look at the book together in the evening when they read it. After a few times the child feels comfortable enough to settle down in bed and just listen to the story on subsequent evenings, and is able to relax even better.

I am often asked how parents should use my books to make bedtime a success. My answer is always to **observe** the child and then **adapt** the story. Here are some questions and answers that give examples of how to observe and adapt the story to every unique child, as well as questions about the books.

I hope these suggestions will help you make the most of my sleep-promoting books. I should emphasise that no-one knows the child as well as you do. This can only be advice for you to bear in mind when you read the book.

My child doesn't like me adding her name in story, it wakes her up.
I would advise you not to say your child's name in a situation like that. Still, most children seem to think it's fun that their name is included in the story, and it makes them more connected with the message of the book.

Sometimes we read to more than one of our children at the same time, should we say all the children's names where it says [Name]?
Try it out. What happens? If they like it, keep doing it; otherwise skip saying the children's names. It's perfectly OK to address the story to one unnamed child, though, because each child will absorb the story into his or her thoughts, so the story will speak specifically to that child.

My child thinks it sounds odd when I emphasize some words or read with a more soothing voice.
One solution is not to emphasize the words so heavily and to read a little more quickly if your child thinks it's going too slowly. You can also read the story normally to start with, without emphasis, or at a more even tempo, and still get your child to relax and feel tired. Try different approaches, and remember to have fun while you're doing so.

I've discovered that my child falls asleep more quickly at a particular part of the book, so I read the same section several times until my child falls asleep. Is that OK?

Absolutely – that's an excellent idea! You can also skip passages or pages if you notice that they somehow stimulate your child.

Do I have to finish the whole story even if my child has fallen asleep already on the second page?

Of course not, as long as you're sure your child really is fast asleep even when you leave the room. A lot of parents have told me that their children sleep more soundly throughout the night after they've listened to the story, so it can be a good idea to keep reading for a while after you think your child has fallen asleep, because it might help him or her to relax even more and reach a wonderful deep sleep.

The book is boring and doesn't stimulate my child's imagination.

My books are not intended to replace the wonderful picture books and chapter books you read with your child. My bedtime stories are specifically for the time when your child needs help to relax and go to sleep, and therefore I don't want the book to be too exciting, as it would have the opposite effect and it will take longer for your child to fall asleep. Even so, I have tried to find a balance where the child's imagination is stimulated by inviting them to imagine things and by including a number of different characters in the books.

I've followed all the advice you've given me, but I still can't get my child to want to listen to the story.

It might be worth trying the audiobook instead, then you can snuggle up together and just listen to the story. Or perhaps try one of the other books in the same series. The books feature different characters and settings that might catch your child's interest long enough for him or her to want to listen to the story and be lulled to sleep. Reading the story is like rocking your child to sleep with words.

For what ages are your sleep-promoting books recommended?

I have received letters saying that everyone from eight-month-old babies to adults with lifelong sleeping problems have managed to fall asleep to my bedtime stories. For that reason, they are not aimed at any specific age. But I do recommend testing and perhaps adapting the content of the story depending on the child's age. For adults, I usually recommend the audiobooks. A lot of people have said those have helped them fall asleep.

SUCCESS FACTORS

Here are some success factors based on what parents have told me after reading the other books in the series, *The Rabbit Who Wants to Fall Asleep* and *The Elephant Who Wants to Fall Asleep:*

- Be persistent
- Create a habit
- Prepare before bedtime
- Focus on relaxation
- Learn from the characters

BE PERSISTENT

Even if your child doesn't fall asleep after you have read the whole story the first time, try reading it again. Give the book a real chance, even reading it through a couple of times. I remember a letter from one family in particular who said that bedtime could take up to five hours each evening. So they started to read *The Rabbit Who Wants to Fall Asleep*. The first evening, they read the whole story two and a half times before their child fell asleep. The following evening, they only needed to read the story once. Over the next few evenings, the length of time shrank further, and by the time they sent their letter, a week or so later, they were down to about eight minutes per evening. Bedtime went from five hours to just eight minutes, thanks to their persistence and faith in the book. Don't give up.

CREATE A HABIT

Read the book several times over a period of time in order to create a habit, which will help your child feel secure enough to relax into the story and want to go to sleep. Parents have told me how *The Rabbit Who Wants to Fall Asleep* has become a natural part of their bedtime routine, that both child and parent know the book by heart, and that the child quickly falls fast asleep each evening. My wife and I had a similar experience with our oldest son. We started playing him the audiobook while he was still in the womb, when we were going to sleep, so he made the mental connection between the story and sleep. After he was born we played the audiobook every evening when it was time to go to sleep. Now he is four years old and falls asleep easily in the evenings, with or without the audiobook, because he has learned to relax. Whenever he's sick or if we're travelling, we use the audiobook to help him feel safe and calm when it's time to go to bed. We now have another child, and are excited to see if the same strategy will help him as well.

PREPARE BEFORE BEDTIME

In order to get the best results with the story, your child should be worn out before you read it. There are, however, examples where parents have said that their very active child has managed to fall fast asleep right at the start of the story. You can also prepare your child before you read the bedtime story by communicating in a special way. Here are a few examples of what you might say:

"You're starting to look tired, even if you might not be aware of it yet."

"It looks like your eyelids are getting heavier and heavier. It'll soon be time to go to sleep."

"You're getting sleepier and sleepier, aren't you? [Yawn]"

"Tonight we're going to read a magical story that will make you want to fall asleep, maybe even before the story ends."

"You know that story we read in the evenings, the one that helps you fall fast asleep? It seems like you're falling asleep quicker and easier each time we read it. That must feel wonderful."

"Tonight I'm going to read a magical story that helps elephants, rabbits, tractors and lovely children like you fall fast asleep."

"You're only allowed to read this magical story when it's time to go to sleep because you're going to end up falling asleep every time we read it."

FOCUS ON RELAXATION

Some parents say that the book is hard to read, or that their child reacts when an adult reads the book in a slightly different way to what they're used to from other books. I'd really like to emphasise that it's perfectly okay to read the book normally, like an ordinary story. It will still have a relaxing effect. Try different approaches to see what works best – both for you and your child. We are all different, of course, and some children will want to look at the pictures while you read the story. If the child is lying down in bed and listening to the story instead of looking at the pictures, it makes the child more focused on what you're saying, making it easier to relax. This is all the more important if you're reading from a tablet or phone, because it's good to avoid the light from the screen, as research has shown that this tends to make children livelier, unless your device have support for night mode.

LEARN FROM THE CHARACTERS

Once you've read one or more of my sleep-promoting books, you and your child will have started to get to know the characters in the books. I strongly believe that you as a parent should talk to your child during the day or evening about what makes the characters go to sleep. They all have different techniques that help them fall asleep. During the conversation you can suggest to the child that he or she might like to try doing what one of the characters does when it's time to go to sleep that evening. Then you can talk about it again at bedtime, and encourage the child to try different things, as a way for him or her to learn to relax and, in the long term, fall asleep without these books.

Good luck with my sleep-promoting books!

Carl-Johan

ABOUT THE BOOK AND THE AUTHOR

Carl-Johan Forssén Ehrlin is a ground-breaking bestselling author whose first children's book, *The Rabbit Who Wants to Fall Asleep*, became a global phenomenon. It was the first self-published book to top Amazon's bestseller list. Thanks to satisfied parents telling their friends about the book and writing about it on social media, word about its magic spread around the world. With more than two million copies sold around the world, *The Rabbit Who Wants to Fall Asleep* is an international success, closely followed by the sequel, *The Little Elephant Who Wants to Fall Asleep*. Today the books have been translated into more than forty-six languages.

The Tractor Who Wants to Fall Asleep is the third book in a series of books, all intended to help children to relax and fall asleep at bedtime.

Carl-Johan Forssén Ehrlin is a professional behavioural expert with a bachelor's degree in psychology, and a certified NLP Master Practitioner. For many years Carl-Johan has been one of Sweden's foremost coaches, lecturers and course directors in the fields of leadership, communication and personal development. Carl-Johan occasionally teaches communication at Jönköping University, and is regularly approached by universities around the world. These days he mostly works as a writer, publishing books in the fields of leadership and personal development as well as books for helping children.

Read more about the author at www.carl-johan.com or follow his Facebook pages *Carl-Johan Forssén Ehrlin* and *The Rabbit Who Wants to Fall Asleep*.

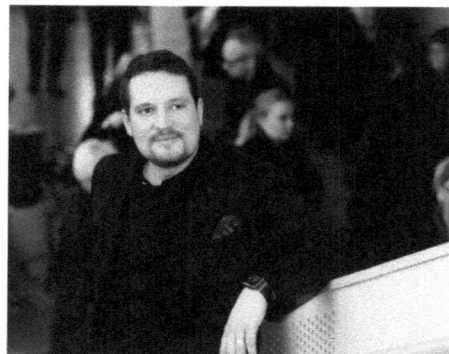

Foto: Jonas Nygren

www.ingramcontent.com/pod-product-compliance
Lightning Source LLC
Chambersburg PA
CBHW040858100426
42813CB00015B/2835